THE *Skinny* SIRT SOUP

Recipe Book

THE SKINNY SIRTFOOD SOUP RECIPE BOOK
DELICIOUS & SIMPLE SIRTFOOD DIET SOUPS FOR HEALTH & WEIGHT LOSS

ISBN 978-1-910771-97-6

A CIP catalogue record of this book is available from the British Library

• •

Disclaimer

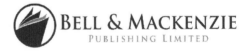
BELL & MACKENZIE
PUBLISHING LIMITED

CONTENTS

VEGETABLE SIRT SOUPS   **45**

CHILLED SIRT SOUPS   **71**

FRUIT SIRT SOUPS

OTHER COOKNATION TITLES

INTRODUCTION

A collection of simple and delicious homemade healthy soup recipes to use as part of your Sirtfood Diet.

Packed full of Sirtuin-rich ingredients, our Sirt soups are the perfect companion to your Sirt diet efforts. All our recipes are easy to prepare, economical and low in calories.

This comprehensive collection includes hearty broths, light fillers, summer soups, vegetarian, seafood and meat options - perfect for speedy lunches and weeknight suppers.

Soup's versatility is what makes it so perfect if you are following the Sirtfood diet. Ingredients can be tailored to make the most of the turbo charging sirtuin-rich foods which can help you lose weight. The healthy, fresh and seasonal ingredients can deliver a protein packed hit, a comforting winter warmer or a light and refreshing consommé.

ABOUT THE SIRTFOOD DIET

The revolutionary Sirtfood diet for weight loss and health - it's about what you CAN eat not what you can't!

A diet that focuses on the positive effects of healthy balanced nutrition, works in perfect tandem with your body, can result in amazing weight loss (up to 7lbs in 7 days), increased energy levels, increased lean muscle, general heightened well being and rarely has you feeling hungry.

You will have likely read the headlines which have highlighted the inclusion and benefits of red wine, coffee and chocolate. Yes it's true they are all on the top list of Sirt-rich foods and can definitely be enjoyed while still losing weight but there are so many other fantastic ingredients and health benefits to focus on when you follow the Sirtfood diet.

If your weight loss efforts in the past have focused on severe calorie restricted diets you'll no doubt be painfully aware that while they can indeed have dramatic slimming results they are also notoriously difficult to sustain. Prolonged calorie restriction/fasting even for two days of the week takes a lot of discipline and often leaves us feeling irritable, tired, hungry and generally miserable. Maintaining this type of diet long term is difficult and many of us fall off the wagon and inevitably end up back where we started often a pound or two heavier and even more demotivated.

So instead of fixating on the negative effects of a diet (e.g. all the foods you CAN'T eat), what if you could diet where the focus was on all the positive foods that you CAN and SHOULD be eating? That's got be good right? The psychological effect on this positive approach is huge in achieving your goals but more than that wouldn't you rather focus on the quality of your food rather than the quantity?

Step forward the Sirtfood Diet. A revolutionary new approach to health and weight loss which has come to the fore thanks to new scientific research which has identified turbocharging foods that activate the 'skinny gene' in all of us.

The science of the Sirtfood diet is fully explained by Aidan Goggins and Glen Matten in their breakthrough book 'The Sirtfood Diet'. Here they trialed their theory based on scientific research on members of one of London's most exclusive health clubs with amazing success. Participants experienced on average 7lbs weight loss in 7 days with increases in lean muscle too. We highly recommend you read their book for a full understanding of the science and research.

To follow is an outline of the Sirtfood diet and how it works backed up with over 70 soup recipes that will compliment your meal plans perfectly.

THE 'SKINNY' GENE

This rather unscientific term relates to a group of genes in our body called sirtuins. Put simply, sirtuins relate to the body's metabolism, insulin and cell repair. Activating these genes is the key to aiding weight loss, making us healthier and living longer.

Research tells us that that there are 2 principal ways to spark theses super genes:

1)   **by restricting calories and exercising**
2)   **by SIRT activators**

We know that restricting calories (a measurement of energy) and expending more energy than we consume (a calorie deficit) will occur in weight loss and this indeed is also part of phase 1 & 2 of the Sirtfood diet.

Q):   So how do we use Sirt activators?

A):   By consuming foods that contain a natural rich source of SIRT activators – also called Sirtfoods.

Sirtfoods activate Sirtuins (the 'skinny' genes) and get to work triggering the body to stop storing fat and instead get its energy, not from primarily glucose, but breaking down the fat stores.

There are seven Sirtuins in the body, named Sirt 1 to Sirt 7, which control metabolism, insulin levels and cell repair. Research continues on the function of these genes but it is known that their activation is a key factor in weight loss, improved health and anti-ageing.

Sirtuins also reduce levels of the hormone IGF-1 (Insulin-like Growth Factor) which is directly responsible for the ageing process. IGF-1 causes the body to grow and produce new cells. By consuming a Sirtfood rich diet, levels of IGF-1 decrease which makes our body focus more on repairing cells which is key to slowing down the ageing process.

WHAT ARE SIRTFOODS?

Sirtfoods are a group of foods rich in special nutrients called polyphenols which when eaten activate sirtuins in our body in the same was as fasting does prompting fat burning while also increasing muscle and levels of cell repair.

Sirtfoods are prevalent in the diets of those with some of the lowest levels of disease and obesity around the world (known as 'blue zones) notably the Kuna American Indians who favour Sirt-rich cocoa in their diet to Okinawa in Japan where a range of nutrient rich Sirtfoods make up much of their daily intake. The well-known Mediterranean diet also contains Sirt-rich food like extra virgin olive oil, nuts, berries, red wine and dates and is key to keeping obesity levels low.

THE TOP SIRTFOODS

There are many foods that contain the powerful sirtuin-activating effects but research has identified the following top foods as being some of the most nutrient rich:

Birds-eye chilli	Red grapes & red wine	Olives & Extra Virgin Olive Oil	Soy & Tofu
Onions	Ground tumeric	Citrus fruits	Dark chocolate & cocoa powder
Buckwheat	Kale	Matcha green tea	

By increasing our daily intake of sirtuin activating foods (Sirtfoods) we can experience all the benefits of the Sirtfood diet – weight loss, more energy, feeling better, maintaining or increasing muscle. Research has also shown that combining Sirt-activating foods with fasting helps regulate appetite in the brain meaning no hunger pangs.

Our recipes combine nutrient packed Sirtfoods with lean protein, omega-rich fish, good carbs and veg to create delicious healthy soups.

MORE SIRTUIN ACTIVATING FOODS

While we've listed the most prolific Sirt-rich foods available there are many others which also pack a good punch of Sirt nutrients which we have incorporated into our soup recipes. Examples of just some of the additional sirtuin activating foods are listed opposite.. We would encourage you to research and seek out as many additional sirtuin activating foods when preparing your own recipes or perhaps to use as a substitute where a top sirtfood ingredient might be missing in your store cupboard.

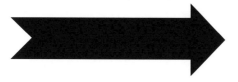

Blackberries	Spinach	Sardines	Coffee
Apples	Asparagus	Trout	Tea
Gogi berries	Cauliflower	Sardines	Fresh apple & orange juice
Blackcurrants	Parsley	Fresh Tuna	Peppermint tea

SIRT PORTIONS

As time moves on you may begin creating your own soup recipes as your Sirt journey continues. As you do start to experiment with your own Sirt cooking it's helpful to know the quantity of each Sirt food you should be using.

Take a look at the quantities of Sirt ingredients we use throughout the recipes in the book to guide you. Very broadly speaking a handful of the listed leaves, greens, and veg constitutes a portion of Sirt food whilst dry spices would be approx. 1 teaspoon and fresh herbs 1 tablespoon.

ABOUT

CookNation is the leading publisher of innovative and practical recipe books for the modern, health conscious cook.

CookNation titles bring together delicious, easy and practical recipes with their unique approach - easy and delicious, no-nonsense recipes - making cooking for diets and healthy eating fast, simple and fun.

With a range of #1 best-selling titles - from the innovative 'Skinny' calorie-counted series, to the 5:2 Diet Recipes collection - CookNation recipe books prove that 'Diet' can still mean 'Delicious'!

Visit **www.bellmackenzie.com** to browse the full catalogue.

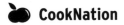

Skinny
SIRT
soup

meat & poultry

SPICED CHICKEN SOUP

398 calories

Ingredients

- 4 medium chicken drumsticks
- 1 red onion, chopped
- 1 carrot, chopped
- 1lt/4 cups chicken stock
- 400g/14oz tinned chopped tomatoes
- 75g/3oz shredded kale
- 250ml/1 cup tomato passata/sieved tomatoes
- 1 green pepper, de-seeded and chopped
- 1 bird's eye chilli, de-seeded & finely chopped

- 2 garlic cloves, crushed
- 1 tsp dried mixed herbs
- 1 tsp paprika
- 1 tsp turmeric
- ½ tsp ground cumin
- 400g/14oz tinned black beans,
- 400g/14oz tinned kidney beans
- 2 tbsp chopped flat leaf parsley
- Salt and freshly ground black pepper

Method

1 Place the onion and carrot in a large saucepan with the chicken drumsticks. Pour over the stock and bring to a simmer. Cook for 20 minutes, then remove the chicken and set to one side.

2 Add the chopped tomatoes, kale, passata, green pepper, chilli & garlic to the pan, and bring back to simmering point. Add the dried herbs, paprika, turmeric & cumin and simmer for 30 minutes.

3 Remove the skin from the drumsticks and pull the chicken off the bone. Shred the chicken meat and return it to the pan. Add the black beans and kidney beans and simmer for a further 6 minutes.

4 Season well and serve with parsley sprinkled over the top.

CHEF'S NOTE
This is a really hearty soup which makes a great evening meal.

BUCKWHEAT MINESTRONE

280 calories

Ingredients

- 1 tbsp extra virgin olive oil
- 1 garlic clove, crushed
- 1 red onion
- 1 celery stalk
- 1 carrot
- 125g/4oz potato
- 2 red peppers, de-seeded
- 200g/7oz kale

- 750ml/3 cups chicken stock
- 1 tsp dried oregano
- 1 tsp dried thyme
- 300g/11oz buckwheat noodles
- 150g/5oz tinned butter beans
- 400g/14oz tomatoes
- 50g/2oz diced pepperoni
- Freshly ground pepper to taste

Method

1 Wash and chop all the fresh vegetables, removing the tough stalks from the kale.

2 Heat the oil in a large saucepan and sauté the chopped onion, garlic, celery, carrot, potato and peppers for a few minutes.

3 Add the stock and dried herbs. Bring to the boil and simmer for 6-8 minutes until the vegetables are tender.

4 Add the butter beans, tomatoes, pepperoni and kale. Return to the boil. Lower the heat and simmer for about 5 minutes, until the kale is just tender. Season with pepper.

5 Add the buckwheat noodles and cook for 2 minutes longer or until tender.

CHEF'S NOTE

Buckwheat noodles are fat free and are a good source of manganese, protein, carbohydrates and thiamine.

ONION & BACON SOUP

SERVES 4

275 calories

Ingredients

- 1 tbsp extra virgin olive oil
- 50g/2oz smoked bacon, finely chopped
- 2 red onions, chopped
- 1 leek, chopped
- 2 garlic cloves, crushed
- 1 tbsp chopped fresh thyme
- 120ml/½ cup red wine
- ½ tsp freshly ground pepper
- 750ml/3 cups chicken stock
- 400g/14oz tinned chickpeas
- 2 tbsp chopped fresh chives

Method

1 Heat the oil in a large saucepan and sauté the onions and bacon until cooked. Add the leek, garlic and thyme and cook, uncovered, stirring often for 3 minutes.

2 Pour in the red wine and add the pepper. Bring to the boil for a moment, reduce the heat and simmer, until most of the red wine has reduced by half.

3 Stir in the stock. Drain and the rinse the chickpeas and add these to the pan. Bring to the boil. Reduce the heat once more and cook for a few minutes until the vegetables are tender.

4 Sprinkle with chives, season are serve.

CHEF'S NOTE
Originally cultivated in the Middle East, chickpeas are also known as garbanzo beans.

CHICKEN, KALE AND SPINACH SOUP

330 calories

Ingredients

- 1 tbsp extra virgin olive oil
- 1 red pepper, de-seeded
- 1 red onion, chopped
- 300g/11oz kale
- 300g/11oz spinach

- 1.25lt/5 cups chicken stock
- 125g/4oz cooked shredded chicken breast
- ½ tsp salt
- 2 tbsp low fat cream cheese
- 2 tbsp finely chopped walnuts

Method

1 Heat the olive oil in a large saucepan and sauté the onion & peppers for a few minutes.

2 Add the kale, spinach, stock & salt, and bring to the boil over medium heat. Reduce the heat and simmer, uncovered, for another 5 minutes or until the kale and spinach are tender.

3 Add the chicken and cream cheese, and warm through for a couple of minutes.

4 Blend the soup until smooth, check the seasoning and serve with walnuts sprinkled over the top.

CHEF'S NOTE
Kale has strong anti-inflammatory properties which are helpful to the body's well being.

CHICKEN AND RADISH SOUP

280 calories

Ingredients

- 3 tbsp extra virgin olive oil
- 2 red onions, chopped
- 6 carrots, chopped
- 50g/2oz radishes, sliced
- 1lt/4 cups chicken stock
- 125g/4oz cooked shredded chicken breast
- 1 tsp sea salt
- 4 tbsp chopped flat leaf parsley
- Salt and black pepper

Method

1 Heat the olive oil in a large saucepan. Sauté the onion for a few minutes, until softened.

2 Add the carrots, radish & stock and bring to the boil. Lower the heat and simmer for half an hour.

3 Blend the soup until smooth. Stir through the chicken and put back on the heat until warmed though.

4 Serve garnished with the parsley and some freshly ground black pepper.

CHEF'S NOTE
Radishes are high in Vitamin C and fibre.

SLOW-COOKED PEA AND HAM SOUP

500 calories

Ingredients

- 450g/1lb ham hock
- 200g/7oz dried green split peas
- 1 red onion, chopped
- 75g/3oz diced carrots
- 225g/8oz chopped celery
- 2 garlic cloves, crushed
- ½ tsp black pepper
- 120ml/½ cup red wine
- 1½lt/6 cups chicken stock
- 2 tbsp chopped flat leaf parsley

Method

1 Put the ham hock in a large slow-cooker. Add all the other ingredients, cover and cook on high for 6 hours until the ham falls off the bone and the split peas are soft.

2 Remove the ham. When it's cool enough to handle, pull the meat off the bone, shred and return to the soup.

3 Divide into bowls, sprinkle with parsley and serve.

CHEF'S NOTE
Cut down cooking time by using bacon instead of ham hock and cooking the soup on the stove top for 20 minutes.

BEEF AND BEETROOT SOUP

390 calories

Ingredients

- 1 tbsp buckwheat flour
- 225g/8oz cubed stewing beef
- 1 tbsp extra virgin olive oil
- 1 red onion, chopped
- 1lt/4 cups chicken or beef stock
- 60ml/¼ cup red wine

- 300g/11oz shredded kale
- 350g/12oz potatoes, peeled and chopped
- 125g/4oz carrots, peeled and chopped
- 225g/8oz beetroot, peeled and chopped
- 4 tbsp low fat crème fraiche
- 4 tbsp flat leaf parsley

Method

1 Place the beef and flour in a plastic bag and shake well to cover the beef pieces.

2 Heat the oil in a large saucepan and tip in the beef. Cook on a high heat, stirring frequently until the meat is browned on all sides.

3 Reduce the heat, stir in the onions and cook for 3 minutes or so until softened. Pour in the stock and the wine, and bring to the boil for a moment. Lower the heat, cover and simmer for 2 hours until the beef is tender.

4 Add the kale, potatoes, carrots and beetroot. Cover again and simmer for another 30 minutes or until the vegetables are tender.

5 Divide into bowls. Garnish with a dollop of crème fraiche and sprinkle with chopped parsley.

CHEF'S NOTE
A sprinkle of paprika over the **crème** fraiche also makes a nice additional garnish.

SPICE BLEND CHICKEN SOUP

290 calories

Ingredients

- 1 red onion, finely chopped
- 1 tbsp extra virgin olive oil
- 2 garlic cloves, crushed
- 2 tsp cumin seeds
- 2 tsp ground coriander/cilantro
- 1 tbsp ground turmeric
- ½ tsp ground cinnamon

- 2 bird's eye chillies, deseeded & finely chopped
- 200g/7oz cooked shredded chicken breast
- 400g/14oz tinned chopped tomatoes
- 1lt/4 cups chicken stock
- 400g/14oz tinned cannellini beans, drained and rinsed

Method

1 Heat the oil in a large saucepan and sauté the onion and garlic over a low heat for a few minutes.

2 Add the cumin, coriander, turmeric, cinnamon and chillies. Add the chicken and stir well.

3 Pour in the chicken stock and chopped tomatoes. Season well and simmer for 20 minutes.

4 Add the cannellini beans and cook for a further 10 minutes.

5 Season and serve.

CHEF'S NOTE
Cumin, coriander & turmeric form a classic spice blend.

VIETNAMESE BUCKWHEAT NOODLE SOUP

466 calories

Ingredients

- 2½lt/10 cups chicken stock
- 1 red onion, sliced into rings
- 1 tsp freshly grated ginger root
- 1 lemongrass stalk
- 1 cinnamon stick
- 1 tsp whole black peppercorns
- 225g/8oz buckwheat noodles
- 400g/14oz beef sirloin steak, very finely sliced
- 175g/6oz bean sprouts
- 1 tbsp chopped fresh basil leaves
- 1 tbsp chopped fresh mint leaves
- 1 tbsp chopped coriander, chopped
- 2 bird's eye chillies, sliced into rings
- 2 limes, cut into wedges
- 2 tbsp soy sauce

Method

1 Pour the stock into a large pan. Add the onion, ginger, lemon grass, cinnamon and peppercorns. Bring to the boil, lower the heat, cover and simmer for 1 hour.

2 Cook the noodles in water until soft. Drain, divide into 4 bowls and set to one side.

3 Add the beef, beansprouts, herbs & chillies to the pan and cook for 1 minute.

4 Divide the soup over the noodles and serve with lime wedges and soy sauce.

CHEF'S NOTE
One minute of cooking will leave the beef slices tender.

WALNUT AND CELERIAC SOUP

395 calories

Ingredients

- 100g/3½oz smoked pancetta, diced
- 1 tbsp extra virgin olive oil
- 1 red onion, chopped
- 1 celeriac bulb, chopped
- 2 celery stalks, sliced
- 150g/5oz potato, finely diced
- 1 bay leaf
- 1lt/4 cups chicken stock
- 2 tbsp chopped walnuts
- 4 tbsp sour cream
- 4 tbsp chopped flat leaf parsley

Method

1 Heat the oil in a large saucepan and fry the pancetta until crispy.

2 Add the onion, celeriac & celery to the pan and sauté for 5 minutes.

3 Add the potato, bay leaf and chicken stock to the pan. Bring to the boil, reduce the heat and simmer for 10-15 minutes until the vegetables are tender.

4 Remove the bay leaf from the soup and blend until smooth.

5 Season and serve with a spoonful of sour cream dolloped in the centre. Sprinkle with walnuts and parsley to serve.

CHEF'S NOTE
Studies have shown celeriac is beneficial for improving immunity, blood production, bone & heart health.

CHORIZO AND CHICORY SOUP

299 calories

Ingredients

- 1 tbsp extra virgin olive oil
- 1 red onion sliced
- 3 garlic cloves, crushed
- 150g/5oz chorizo, diced
- ½ tsp cumin seeds
- 200g/7oz red chicory, shredded
- 200g/7oz Savoy cabbage, thinly shredded
- 400g/14oz tinned chopped tomatoes
- 1lt/4 cups chicken stock
- 4 tbsp low fat crème fraîche
- 2 tbsp chopped flat leaf parsley

Method

1 Heat the olive oil in a large saucepan and gently sauté the onion & garlic for a few minutes.

2 Add the chorizo and cumin seeds and cook for a few minutes longer.

3 Add the chicory, cabbage, stock & tomatoes. Increase the heat and simmer for 20 minutes, stirring occasionally.

4 Remove from the heat. Stir through the crème fraiche, sprinkle with chopped parsley and serve.

CHEF'S NOTE
Red chicory contains luteolin which neutralizes free radicals and helps reduce inflammation.

CHICKEN MULLIGATAWNY

330 calories

Ingredients

- 75g/3oz cooked brown rice
- 1 tbsp extra-virgin olive oil
- 1 red onion, finely chopped
- 1 stalk celery, chopped
- 1 carrot, diced
- 1 parsnip, diced
- 125g/4oz potato, diced
- 1 red pepper, de-seeded and chopped
- 1 bird's eye chilli, de-seeded and finely sliced
- 1 tbsp medium curry paste
- 1 tsp turmeric powder
- 370ml/1½ cups tomato passata/sieved tomatoes
- 750ml/3 cups chicken stock
- 300g/11oz cooked shredded chicken breast
- Salt and pepper to season

Method

1 Cook the rice in boiling water until tender, drain and set to one side.

2 Meanwhile heat the oil in a large pan and sauté the onion for 5 minutes. Add the celery, carrot, parsnip, potato, red pepper & chilli and cook for a few minutes more.

3 Stir through the curry paste, turmeric and passata. Add the stock and simmer for 10 minutes until the vegetables are tender.

4 Add the cooked rice and chicken, and cook for a couple of minutes until everything is piping hot.

5 Season and serve.

CHEF'S NOTE
The soup can be frozen and kept for up to 3 months.

IRISH LAMB & KALE SOUP

410 calories

Ingredients

- 2 tbsp extra-virgin olive oil
- 400g/14oz lamb fillet, trimmed & cubed
- 2 red onions, sliced
- 2 leeks, thickly sliced
- 1lt/4 cups vegetable stock
- 250g/9oz potatoes, peeled and chopped
- 1 carrot, thickly sliced
- 200g/7oz kale, chopped
- 400g/14oz tinned chopped tomatoes
- 2 tbsp tomato puree/paste
- 1 tsp dried thyme
- 2 tbsp chopped fresh flat leaf parsley

Method

1 Heat the oil in a large saucepan on a high heat and brown the cubes of lamb for a few minutes.

2 Remove the browned lamb from the pan. Add the onions and cook gently sauté for a few minutes until golden.

3 Return the lamb to the pan. Add the leeks & stock and bring to the boil.

4 Lower the heat and simmer gently, covered, for about 1 hour, stirring occasionally.

5 Add the potatoes, carrot, kale, tinned tomatoes, puree & thyme to the pan and gently simmer for 30 minutes, until the lamb is very tender.

6 Use a fork to shred the lamb before serving.

CHEF'S NOTE
Use the leanest cut of lamb possible otherwise you may need to skim any additional fat from the soup surface before serving.

BACON AND WATERCRESS SOUP

297 calories

Ingredients

- 50g/2oz smoked back bacon
- 2 tbsp extra virgin olive oil
- 1 red onion, chopped
- 1 garlic clove, crushed
- 150g/5oz potato, cubed
- 1lt/4 cups chicken stock
- 400g/14oz frozen peas
- 75g/3oz kale, shredded
- 75g/3oz watercress
- 2 tbsp chopped flat leaf parsley
- Salt and black pepper

Method

1 First cook the bacon in the olive oil for a few minutes until crispy. Remove from the pan, finely chop and set to one side.

2 Reduce the heat and sauté the onion and garlic (in the same pan as the bacon) for a few minutes until softened. Add the potato and stock. Increase the heat and simmer for 15 minutes, until the potatoes are tender.

3 Add the peas, kale & watercress and simmer for a further 3 minutes.

4 Place in a blender and blend until smooth. Season to taste with salt and freshly ground black pepper.

5 Serve the soup with the chopped bacon and parsley sprinkled over the top.

CHEF'S NOTE
Watercress, kale & spinach combine together to make a super green SIRT combination.

MUTTON BROTH

405 calories

Ingredients

- 1 tbsp extra virgin olive oil
- 1 red onion, sliced
- 400g/14oz mutton, cubed
- 50g/2oz pearl barley, pre-soaked
- 50g/2oz split peas, pre-soaked
- 1 leek, sliced

- 175g/6oz kale
- 1½lt/6 cups vegetable stock
- 200g/7oz carrots, chopped
- 2 tbsp chopped fresh flat leaf parsley
- Salt and pepper
- 75g/3oz Savoy cabbage

Method

1 Heat the oil in a large pan and sauté the onion for a few minutes until softened.

2 Add, the stock and mutton. Simmer for 30 minutes, then add the barley & peas and simmer for another 30 minutes.

3 Take the pan off the heat. Shred the meat. Skim any fat from the surface of the soup. Return the mutton to the pan along with all the other ingredients.

4 Simmer for another 20 minutes, or until the vegetables are tender.

5 Season with salt and pepper and serve.

CHEF'S NOTE
Mutton adds a gamey taste. It can be a little fatty so make sure you use a lean cut.

RED ONION SOUP

250 calories

Ingredients

- 2 tbsp extra virgin olive oil
- 75g/3oz chorizo, finely chopped
- 600g/1lb 5oz red onions, finely sliced
- 3 garlic cloves, crushed
- 400g/14oz tinned chopped tomatoes

- 1 tbsp balsamic vinegar
- 1 tsp dried thyme
- 250ml/1 cup red wine
- 500ml/2 cups chicken stock
- Salt and pepper

Method

1 Heat the oil in a large saucepan. Add the chorizo & onion and cook slowly on low heat for about half an hour, stirring occasionally.

2 When the onions are soft, add the tomatoes, balsamic vinegar, garlic & thyme. Cover and simmer for 15 minutes.

3 Add the wine, turn up the heat and boil until the liquid is reduced by about half.

4 Pour in the stock, bring back to the boil, and simmer for another 30 minutes.

5 Season and serve.

CHEF'S NOTE
Onions have been used as a preventative cure for colds dating back to Roman times.

KALE AND RED WINE SOUP

280 calories

Ingredients

- 1 tbsp extra virgin olive oil
- 1 red onion, sliced
- 4 garlic cloves, crushed
- 1 tbsp fresh chopped oregano
- 1 tbsp fresh chopped basil
- 250ml/1 cup red wine

- 1lt/4 cups chicken stock
- 800g/1¾lb tinned chopped tomatoes
- 50g/2oz buckwheat pasta
- 175g/6oz kale, rinsed, stems removed
- 2 tbsp balsamic vinegar
- 2 tbsp fresh chopped flat leaf parsley

Method

1 Heat the oil in a large saucepan. Sauté the onion and garlic for a few minutes until softened. Stir in the oregano, basil and wine. Add the tomatoes and pour in the stock. Bring to the boil.

2 Add the buckwheat pasta, lower the heat and simmer for 10 minutes, until the pasta is tender.

3 Stir in the kale and balsamic vinegar and cook for a further 5 minutes or so until it's wilted.

4 Season and serve with parsley sprinkled over the top.

CHEF'S NOTE
Use really small buckwheat pasta shapes or break op some buckwheat noodles into little pieces.

COCONUT AND BEEF CURRY SOUP

390 calories

Ingredients

- 1 tbsp extra virgin olive oil
- 2 small peppers, de-seeded & chopped
- 1 red onion, chopped
- 3 garlic cloves, crushed
- 2 tsp freshly grated ginger
- 750ml/3 cups beef or chicken stock
- 1½ tbsp soy sauce
- 1½ tbsp rice vinegar
- 1 tbsp brown sugar
- 1 tsp fish sauce
- 1 tsp ground coriander/cilantro
- 1 bird's eye chilli, de-seeded & chopped
- 1 tsp turmeric
- Salt and black pepper to taste
- 250ml/1 cup light coconut milk
- 300g/11oz beef steak, very thinly sliced
- 2 tbsp chopped fresh flat leaf parsley

Method

1 Heat the oil in a large pan and gently sauté the peppers, onion, garlic & ginger for a few minutes until the onions soften.

2 Add the stock, soy sauce, rice vinegar, sugar, fish sauce, coriander, chilli and turmeric. Season with salt and pepper. Increase the heat and simmer for 10 minutes.

3 Add the beef slices and cook for one minute. Stir through the coconut milk & parsley.

4 Serve immediately.

CHEF'S NOTE
Cooking the beef for just one minute will leave it tender and juicy.

BEAN & RICE SOUP

370 calories

Ingredients

- 2 tbsp extra virgin olive oil
- 1 red onion, chopped
- 1 large celery stalk, chopped
- 1 medium green pepper, de-seeded & chopped
- 2 garlic cloves, crushed
- 1 bird's eye chilli, de-seeded & sliced
- 1 tsp ground cumin

- 1 tsp turmeric
- 800g/1¾lb haricot beans, rinsed & drained
- 750ml/3 cups chicken stock
- 1 tbsp tomato puree/paste
- 125g/4oz cooked brown rice
- 125g/4oz cooked chicken breast, finely shredded

Method

1 Heat the oil in a large saucepan and gently sauté the onion, celery, pepper and garlic for a few minutes until softened.

2 Add the chilli, cumin & turmeric, and stir for another minute.

3 Add the beans, stock and tomato puree, and simmer for 20 minutes. When it's cooked use a fork to gently mash some of the beans together to create a thick base for the soup.

4 Divide into bowls, top with the cooked rice & chicken and serve.

CHEF'S NOTE
For varied texture, mash only part of the bean mixture, leaving the rest whole.

CHICKEN & ROCKET SOUP

348 calories

Ingredients

- 1lt/4 cups chicken stock
- 1 red onion, chopped
- 2 large carrots, chopped
- 3 celery stalks , chopped
- 1 garlic clove, crushed
- 500g/1lb 2oz cooked shredded chicken breast
- 4 tbsp fresh chopped flat parsley
- 75g/3oz rocket
- Salt and black pepper

Method

1 Place the stock, onion, carrots, celery and garlic in a large pan. Bring to the boil and simmer for 10 minutes or until the carrots are tender.

2 Blend the soup until smooth and return to the pan. Stir through the chicken breast & parsley and warm through for a minute or two.

3 Divide the soup into bowls, season, pile the rocket on top and serve.

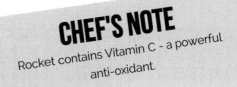

CHEF'S NOTE
Rocket contains Vitamin C - a powerful anti-oxidant.

LOVAGE AND CHICKEN SOUP

298 calories

Ingredients

- 2 tbsp extra virgin olive oil
- 1 leek, chopped
- 1 red onion, chopped
- 1lt/4 cups chicken stock
- 300g/11oz potatoes, chopped
- 50g/2oz lovage leaves
- Sea salt and black pepper
- 300g/11oz cooked shredded chicken breast
- 4 tbsp low fat crème fraiche

Method

1 Heat the oil in a large saucepan and gently sauté the leek & onion for a few minutes until tender.

2 Add the stock and potatoes. Increase the heat and simmer for 10 minutes or until the potatoes are tender.

3 Stir in the lovage leaves and simmer for 5 minutes.

4 Blend the soup until smooth and return to the pan. Stir through the chicken breast and warm through for a minute or two.

5 Check the seasoning, divide the soup into bowls, dollop a tablespoon of crème fraiche in the centre and serve.

CHEF'S NOTE

Also known as sea parsley, lovage adds an intense celery-like flavour to soups.

Skinny
SIRT
soup

seafood

CAPER & RED WINE FISH SOUP

395 calories

Ingredients

- 4 tbsp extra virgin olive oil
- 250g/9oz new potatoes, quartered
- 275g/10oz salmon fillet, diced
- 225g/8oz scallops
- 2 red onions, chopped
- 4 tsp mixed herbs
- 1 bird's eye chillies, de-seeded & chopped
- ½ tsp sea salt
- ½ tsp freshly ground black pepper
- 250ml/1 cup red wine
- 500ml/2 cups fish stock
- 6 ripe plum tomatoes, diced
- 4 tbsp capers, rinsed
- 4 tbsp chopped flat leaf parsley

Method

1 Boil the potatoes for 8-10 minutes or until just tender. Drain and set to one side.

2 Meanwhile chop the salmon into chunks. Heat half the olive oil in a large pan and cook the salmon chunks for a couple of minutes until they begin turning opaque. Transfer to a plate and set to one side.

3 Add the remaining oil to the pan and sauté the red onions for a few minutes. Add the chopped chilli, mixed herbs, salt & pepper and cook for a minute or two longer.

4 Add the wine, stock and tomatoes and bring to the boil.. Reduce heat and cook, stirring often for 5 minutes.

5 Rinse the capers and add these along with the salmon, scallops and potatoes. Return the pan to a simmer and cook for a further 2 minutes. Garnish with fresh chopped parsley.

CHEF'S NOTE
Salmon is one a good source of vitamins B6 & B12.

COD CHOWDER

261 calories

Ingredients

- 2 tbsp extra virgin olive oil
- 1 onion, chopped
- 4 celery stalks, chopped
- 50g/2oz buckwheat flour
- 2 tsp Worcestershire sauce
- ¾ tsp mixed spice
- 750ml/3 cups fish stock
- 250ml/1 cup skimmed milk
- 450g/1lb potatoes, peeled & diced
- 225g/8oz green beans
- 350g/12oz cod fillets, cut into 2cm pieces
- 4 tbsp chopped flat leaf parsley
- Salt and black pepper

Method

1 Heat the oil in a large saucepan and sauté the onion and celery for 5 minutes, until softened. Stir through the buckwheat flour, Worcestershire sauce, and mixed spice.

2 Add the fish stock & milk, and bring to the boil, stirring constantly. Stir in potatoes and green beans, and reduce the heat. Simmer uncovered, stirring occasionally for 10-15 minutes, until the potatoes are cooked.

3 Add the cod and cook, for 4-5 minutes or until the fish is cooked through and easily flakes with a fork.

4 Season well and serve with parsley sprinkled over the top.

CHEF'S NOTE
Try using the back of a fork to gently crush some of the potatoes during cooking to make a thicker base for the soup.

PRAWN & BUCKWHEAT NOODLE SOUP

299 calories

Ingredients

- 1 tbsp extra virgin olive oil
- 3 garlic cloves, crushed
- 1 red onion, finely chopped
- 300g/11oz kale, finely shredded, stems removed
- 1lt/4 cups fish stock
- 300g/11oz small prawns, shelled
- 4 tbsp soy sauce
- 2 tbsp red wine vinegar
- 125g/4oz buckwheat noodles

Method

1 Heat the oil in a large saucepan over medium heat and sauté the garlic and onions for a few minutes until softened.

2 Add the kale, stock, prawns, soy sauce & vinegar. Return to a simmer and cook for 2 minutes.

3 Add the noodles to the pan and cook for further 2-4 minutes or until the prawns are cooked through and the noodles are tender.

4 Season and serve.

CHEF'S NOTE
Shredded pak choi/bok choi instead of kale works equally well in this tasty soup.

WATERCRESS & TILAPIA SOUP

242 calories

Ingredients

- 225g/8oz brown rice
- Zest and juice of 1 lemon
- 1lt/4 cups vegetable stock
- 450g/1lb tilapia fillets, cubed
- 75g/3oz watercress, tough stems removed
- 50g/2oz grated carrot
- 4 tbsp chopped flat leaf parsley
- 1 red onion, finely chopped

Method

1 Cook the rice in a pan of boiling water until tender. Drain, stir through the lemon juice & zest and put to one side.

2 Meanwhile cook the fish in the stock for a few minutes or until it is cooked through and can be easily flaked with a fork.

3 Add the rice to the fish in the pan, warm through quickly and divide into bowls.

4 Roughly chop the watercress and pile this along with the grated carrots, parsley and chopped onions on the top of each bowl. Serve immediately.

CHEF'S NOTE
Watercress has a lovely peppery quality and actually contains more vitamin C than oranges.

CAULIFLOWER & SALMON SOUP

220 calories

Ingredients

- 1 tbsp extra virgin olive oil
- 1 medium carrot, chopped
- 1 celery stalk, chopped
- ½ red onion, finely chopped
- 300g/11oz potatoes, peeled & finely diced
- 1lt/4 cups chicken or fish stock

- 275g/10oz salmon fillet, cubed
- 200g/7oz cauliflower, roughly chopped
- 2 tsp dried tarragon
- 1 tbsp Dijon mustard
- Salt and black pepper
- 4 tbsp chopped flat leaf parsley

Method

1 Heat the oil in a large saucepan and gently sauté the carrot, celery, onion & potatoes for 5-8 minutes or until they begin to go a little soft.

2 Add the stock, salmon & cauliflower and gently simmer for 5 to 7 minutes or until the salmon is just cooked through.

3 Gently stir through the tarragon and mustard.

4 Season with salt and pepper and serve with parsley sprinkled over the top.

CHEF'S NOTE
Make sure the potatoes are finely diced (less the 1cm cubes). This means they'll cook quickly and will give a base to the soup.

ORIENTAL SEAFOOD SOUP

340 calories

Ingredients

- 2 tbsp extra-virgin olive oil
- 1 red onion, chopped
- 2 garlic cloves, crushed
- 1 tbsp grated fresh ginger
- Juice and zest of 1 lime
- 1 bird's eye chilli, de-seeded & thinly sliced
- 1½ tbsp buckwheat flour

- 1lt/4 cups chicken or fish stock
- 175g/6oz cod fillet, cubed
- 300g/11oz small prawns, peeled & chopped
- 5 large shiitake mushroom caps, sliced
- ½ ripe avocado, peeled and diced
- 2 tbsp chopped fresh coriander/cilantro

Method

1 Heat the oil in a large saucepan. Sauté the red onion, garlic, ginger, lime zest and chilli for a few minutes until softened.

2 Stir in the flour and add the stock. Keep stirring while you bring the pan to the boil. Reduce the heat to a simmer and cook for 10 minutes.

3 Add the fish, prawns & mushrooms to the soup. Return to a gentle simmer for about 3 or 4 minutes until the seafood is cooked through.

4 Remove the pan from the heat and stir in the lime juice.

5 Divide into bowls and serve garnished with the cubed avocado pieces and coriander leaves.

CHEF'S NOTE
Prawns are a great source of high quality protein, and provide some of the most important vitamins and minerals that make up a healthy diet.

HOT LIME AND SHRIMP SOUP

104 calories

Ingredients

- 1lt/4 cups fish or chicken stock
- 1 red onion, peeled & quartered
- 2 bird's eye chillies, de-seeded and quartered
- 8 garlic cloves, crushed
- Juice and zest from 1 lime
- ½ tsp cumin seeds
- 1 cinnamon stick
- 450g/1lb prawns, peeled and chopped
- ½ tsp salt
- 2 tbsp each of chopped coriander & flat leaf parsley

Method

1 Add the stock, red onion, chillies, garlic, lime zest, cumin seeds & cinnamon stick to a saucepan.

2 Bring to the boil, reduce the heat, cover and simmer for 20 minutes.

3 Strain the soup and return only the liquid to the pan. Bring to a low simmer. Add the prawns, lime juice and salt. Cook for about 3 minutes, until the prawns are pink and cooked through.

4 Stir through the fresh herbs and serve.

CHEF'S NOTE
Limes contain active compounds called flavonol glycosides which have antioxidant benefits.

MEDITERRANEAN SEA BASS SOUP

240 calories

Ingredients

- 1 red onion, chopped
- 2 celery stalks, chopped
- 2 garlic cloves, crushed
- 1 tbsp extra virgin olive oil
- 250ml/1 cup fish or chicken stock
- 60ml/¼ cup red wine
- 400g/14oz tinned chopped tomatoes
- 250ml/1 cup tomato passata/sieved tomatoes
- 2 tsp dried oregano
- 225g/8oz sea bass fillets, cubed
- 175g/6oz prawns, peeled and chopped
- 1 handful black olives, sliced
- Salt and black pepper
- 2 tbsp fresh chopped flat leaf parsley

Method

1 Heat the oil in large saucepan, and sauté the onion, celery, and garlic until soft. Stir in the stock and the wine. Bring to the boil, lower the heat and simmer for 5 minutes, uncovered.

2 Add the tinned tomatoes, tomato passata and oregano. Season well and simmer for 5 minutes.

3 Gently stir in the sea bass, prawns & sliced olives. Cover and simmer for 3 to 5 minutes or until the fish flakes easily with a fork and the prawns are cooked through.

4 Serve sprinkled with parsley.

CHEF'S NOTE

Use any kind of firm white fish you prefer in place of sea bass.

FISH AND RED WINE SOUP

360 calories

Ingredients

- 750ml/3 cups red wine
- 450g/1lb white fish fillets
- 1 red onion, chopped
- 1 tbsp extra virgin olive oil
- 800g/1¾lb tinned chopped tomatoes
- 4 tbsp chopped flat leaf freshly parsley
- Salt and pepper

Method

1 Place the fish fillets flat in a large frying pan. Pour the wine over and bring to the boil. Reduce the heat and simmer for about 5 minutes, turning at least once.

2 When the fish is cooked through, flake the fillets with a fork. Remove them from the wine with a slotted spoon and set aside.

3 Heat the olive oil in a separate pan, and sauté the onions until soft. Add them to the wine, along with the tinned tomatoes and parsley.

4 Turn up the heat and boil vigorously for at least 10 minutes. Lower the heat again, and add the cooked fish pieces to heat through again. Season well and serve.

CHEF'S NOTE
Use the best quality tinned tomatoes you can get your hands on.

HEARTY SOUP

370 calories

Ingredients

- 2 sprigs parsley
- 2 sprigs thyme
- 1 bay leaf
- 1 celery stalk, chopped
- 400g/14oz tinned chopped tomatoes
- 750ml/3 cups fish stock
- 4 tbsp red wine
- 1 red onion, chopped
- 400g/14oz potatoes, peeled and diced

- 225g/8oz carrots, thickly sliced
- 225g/8oz courgettes, thickly sliced
- 1 red pepper, de-seeded and chopped
- 550g/1¼lb cod fillet, cubed
- Salt and pepper
- 2 tbsp chopped flat leaf parsley
- 1 tbsp chopped chives
- Grated zest of 1 lemon

Method

1 Tie the parsley, thyme and bay leaf and celery together with cotton to make a bouquet garni.

2 Add this along with the tomatoes, stock, red wine and onion. Stir and bring to the boil. Reduce heat and simmer for 15 minutes.

3 Add the potatoes and carrots. Turn up the heat and cook, covered, for another 10 minutes until the potatoes are becoming tender. Stir in the courgettes and red pepper. Cover the pan again and simmer for 5 minutes or until all the vegetables are cooked.

4 Remove the bouquet garni. Add the cod, cover and cook gently for about 5 minutes until the fish is cooked through and flakes easily with a fork.

5 Divide into bowls. Sprinkle over the parsley, chives & zest and serve.

CHEF'S NOTE
Use the seasoning to balance the acidity of the chopped tomatoes.

SPICY MIXED SEAFOOD SOUP

360 calories

Ingredients

- 1 tbsp extra virgin olive oil
- 50g/2oz smoked bacon, chopped
- 1 red onion, chopped
- 1 garlic clove, crushed
- 1 bird's eye chilli, de-seeded & finely chopped
- 1 tbsp buckwheat flour
- 750ml/3 cups fish stock
- 200g/7oz potatoes, peeled & diced
- 175ml/¾ cup skimmed milk
- Salt & pepper
- 400g/14oz white fish fillets, cubed
- 225g/8oz mixed shellfish
- 4 tbsp chopped fresh flat leaf parsley
- 4 tbsp crème fraiche

Method

1 Heat the oil in a large saucepan and fry the bacon until evenly browned. Add the onion, garlic and chilli and cook for another 3 minutes until soft.

2 Stir in the buckwheat flour and cook for a minute or two. Add the fish stock, potatoes & milk, season well and simmer for around 10 minutes or until the potatoes are cooked.

3 Add to the soup, and simmer gently for 5 minutes. Add the fish fillets and mixed shellfish to the soup and cook for a few minutes until the seafood is cooked through.

4 Divide into bowls, add a dollop of crème fraiche, sprinkle over the parsley and serve.

CHEF'S NOTE
Leave out the bacon if you don't want to use meat in your soup.

Skinny
SIRT
soup

vegetable

CURRIED COCONUT AND SQUASH SOUP

300 calories

Ingredients

- 1 tbsp extra-virgin olive oil
- 1 red onion, chopped
- 1 tbsp fresh grated root ginger
- 3 garlic cloves, crushed
- 1 tbsp red curry paste
- 2 tsp turmeric
- 800g/¾lbs butternut squash flesh, chopped
- 750ml/3 cups vegetable stock
- 125g/4oz potato, chopped
- 1 tsp brown sugar
- Salt and pepper
- 2 tbsp fresh lime juice
- 250ml/1 cup light coconut milk
- 2 tbsp fresh chopped flat leaf parsley

Method

1 Heat the oil in a saucepan, and gently sauté the onion, ginger, garlic, and curry paste for a few minutes until softened.

2 Add the turmeric, squash, stock, potato & sugar and simmer for 20 minutes.

3 Blend until smooth. Stir in the lime juice and coconut milk and serve with the sprinkled parsley over the top.

CHEF'S NOTE
Butternut squash contains many vital poly-phenolic anti-oxidants and vitamins.

CREAM OF TOMATO SOUP

268 calories

Ingredients

- 2 red onions
- 1 celery stalk
- 3 tbsp extra virgin olive oil
- 1½ tbsp buckwheat flour
- 250ml/1 cup low fat single cream
- 400g/14oz tinned tomatoes
- 750ml/3 cups vegetable stock
- 3 tbsp freshly chopped rosemary leaves
- 3 tbsp tomato purée
- 1 tbsp soy sauce
- Sea salt and pepper

Method

1 Roughly chop the onions and celery. Heat the oil in a saucepan over a low heat and sauté the onions and celery until slightly softened.

2 Stir in the flour then slowly pour in the cream, stirring all the time until smooth.

3 Add the chopped tomatoes a little at a time, stirring well. Gradually stir in the vegetable stock.

4 Add the rosemary, tomato purée & soy sauce, and season with salt and pepper to taste. Bring the soup to a simmer and cook for 5 more minutes, then blend until smooth. Serve.

CHEF'S NOTE

If you have the time, use fresh tomatoes instead of tinned.

SUPER GREEN SOUP

EXCELLENT ✓ ****

143 calories

Ingredients

- 4 garlic cloves
- 1 tsp fresh ginger
- 400g/14oz courgettes
- 175g/6oz broccoli
- 200g/7oz kale
- 2 tbsp extra virgin olive oil
- 1 tsp ground coriander/cilantro
- 1 tsp ground turmeric
- Pinch sea salt
- 3 tbsp water
- 1lt/4 cups vegetable stock
- 1 lime
- 3 tbsp fresh chopped flat leaf parsley

Method

1 Peel and slice the garlic gloves and ginger. Wash and roughly chop the courgettes, broccoli and kale, making sure to cut out the kale's thick stalks. Juice the lime and grate off the zest.

2 Heat the oil in a large pan. Sauté the garlic & ginger along with the coriander and turmeric for about 2 minutes. Add the salt and the water.

3 Stir in the courgettes, and continue cooking for 3-4 minutes. Add the stock and simmer for another 3 minutes.

4 Add the broccoli, kale and lime juice. Leave to cook again for another 5-7 minutes, until all the vegetables are soft.

5 Remove the pan from the heat and add the chopped parsley. Blend until the soup is smooth.

6 Serve garnished with lime zest.

CHEF'S NOTE
For a thinner soup, use less stock.

EASY VEGETABLE SOUP

225 calories

Ingredients

- 2 red onions
- 3 celery stalks
- 125g/4oz carrots
- 450g/1lb potatoes

- 2 tbsp extra virgin olive oil
- 1lt/4 cups vegetable stock
- 2 tbsp crème fraîche
- 3 tbsp freshly chopped flat leaf parsley

Method

1 Peel and chop all the vegetables and potatoes.

2 Heat the oil in a large saucepan, and sauté the vegetables and potatoes for a few minutes until they begin to soften.

3 Pour in the stock and bring to the boil. Cover and simmer for 15 minutes until the vegetables are all tender.

4 Blend until smooth, then season to taste.

5 Serve with a teaspoon of crème fraîche dolloped in the middle and a good sprinkling of parsley.

CHEF'S NOTE
This soup can be frozen for up to a month.

SPICY VEGETABLE SOUP

243 calories

Ingredients

- 1 red onion
- 2 garlic cloves
- 300g/11oz carrot
- 300g/11oz parsnip
- 300g/11oz peeled butternut squash
- 100g/3½oz potato
- 1 tbsp turmeric

- 2 tsp ras el hanout blended spice
- 1 tbsp extra virgin olive oil
- 1.25lt/5 cups vegetable stock
- 4 tbsp Greek-style yogurt
- 1 tbsp finely chopped mint
- Salt & pepper to season

Method

1 Pre-heat the oven to 200C/180C fan/gas mark 6.

2 Peel the onion and garlic. Cut the onion into about 8 rough wedges. Wash and roughly chop all the other vegetables into 2cm chunks and place in a roasting tin with the onion and garlic cloves.

3 Sprinkle over the turmeric and ras el hanout spice blend. Season. Drizzle over the olive oil and stir well.

4 Roast for half an hour, turning the vegetables halfway through cooking.

5 Transfer the roasted vegetables to a large saucepan. Pour in the stock and simmer for 5-10 minutes until everything is tender. Blend the soup until smooth.

6 Serve with a spoonful of yogurt, and a little chopped mint.

CHEF'S NOTE
Ras el hanout is a North African medley of fragrant spices.

EASY MOROCCAN TOMATO SOUP

248 calories

Ingredients

- 1 red onion
- 2 stalks celery
- 1 clove garlic
- 1 tbsp olive oil
- 1 tsp ground cumin
- 1 tsp ground turmeric
- 750ml/3 cups vegetable stock
- 400g/14oz tinned chopped tomatoes
- 400g/14oz tinned chickpeas, rinsed and drained
- Black pepper
- 100g/3½oz frozen broad beans
- ½ lemon, zest and juice
- 2 tbsp each chopped coriander and flat leaf parsley

Method

1 Peel and chop the onion. Wash and chop the celery. Peel and crush the garlic.

2 Heat the oil in a large saucepan and sauté the onion, garlic and celery gently until softened. Add the cumin and turmeric and stir for another minute.

3 Add the stock, tomatoes and chickpeas & freshly ground black pepper to taste. Bring to the boil & simmer for about 8 minutes.

4 Add the broad beans and lemon juice then cook for a further 2 minutes or so. Season to taste.

5 Serve with a sprinkling of lemon zest, chopped parsley and coriander.

CHEF'S NOTE
Tasty on its own or with buckwheat flatbread.

HOT PUMPKIN SOUP

280 calories

Ingredients

- 1kg/2¼lb pumpkin
- 1 red onion, sliced
- 2 tbsp extra virgin olive oil
- 1 tbsp grated fresh ginger
- 1 lemongrass stalk
- 2 tbsp Thai red curry paste
- 300ml coconut milk
- 750ml/3 cups vegetable stock
- Juice of ½ lime
- 1 bird's eye chilli, de-seeded & very finely sliced

Method

1 Pre-heat the oven to 200C/180C fan/gas 6.

2 Peel and roughly chop the pumpkin. Peel and slice the onion.

3 Toss the pumpkin in a roasting tin with half the oil and season well. Roast for 30 mins, until golden.

4 Meanwhile, heat the remaining oil in a large pan. Add the sliced red onion, ginger and lemongrass. Gently cook for about 10 minutes until softened. Stir the curry paste in well.

5 Tip the roasted pumpkin into the pan. Reserve 3 tbsp of the coconut milk, and add the rest to the pan along with the vegetable stock.

6 Bring to the boil, then reduce the heat and simmer for 5 minutes. Remove the lemongrass stalk, and blend the soup until smooth. Add the lime juice and season to taste.

7 Serve drizzled with the remaining coconut milk and sprinkled with the finely sliced chilli.

CHEF'S NOTE

This soup works well with any kind of squash.

BUTTERNUT SQUASH SOUP

240 calories

Ingredients

- 1 large red onion
- 1kg/2¼lb butternut squash
- 2 tbsp extra virgin olive oil

- 250ml/1 cup red wine
- 750ml/3 cups vegetable stock
- 3 tbsp chopped flat leaf parsley

Method

1 Peel and quarter the onion. Peel, de-seed and roughly chop the squash.

2 Heat the olive oil in a large saucepan and sauté the onion until softened.

3 Add the wine and squash and cook for a couple of minutes before adding the stock and half of the parsley. Bring to the boil, cover and simmer for about 20 minutes or until the squash is tender.

4 Blend until smooth. Serve garnished with the remaining parsley.

CHEF'S NOTE
This soup will keep in the fridge for 2 days, or in the freezer for 6 weeks.

CAULIFLOWER SOUP

318 calories

Ingredients

- 675g/1½lbs cauliflower
- 75g/3oz kale
- 3 stalks celery
- 1 leek
- 1 parsnip
- 3 tbsp extra virgin olive oil
- 1 garlic clove, crushed
- 1 tsp chopped rosemary

- 1 tsp chopped thyme
- 1 tbsp chopped flat leaf parsley
- 500ml/2 cups low fat coconut milk
- 500ml/2 cups vegetable stock
- 1 tsp sea salt
- Black pepper
- Pinch of ground nutmeg

Method

1 Wash and roughly chop the cauliflower, kale, celery, leek and parsnip. Make sure you cut out the thick stalks from the kale.

2 Heat the oil in a large saucepan, and sauté the chopped vegetables, along with the garlic, rosemary and thyme.

3 After a few minutes, add the stock and coconut milk. Bring to the boil and simmer for around 20 minutes.

4 Blend the soup until smooth then season with salt, pepper and nutmeg to taste.

CHEF'S NOTE
Garnish with more fresh parsley to further boost your Sirt intake.

LENTIL AND SQUASH SOUP

240 calories

Ingredients

- 2 red onions
- 300g/11oz butternut squash flesh
- 1lt/4 cups vegetable stock
- 140g/4½oz red lentils
- 3 garlic cloves, crushed
- 1 tsp ground cumin
- 1 tsp ground turmeric
- Pinch cayenne pepper
- 1 tbsp chopped coriander/cilantro
- 1 tbsp chopped flat leaf parsley
- 1 tbsp lemon juice
- Salt and black pepper

Method

1 Peel and roughly chop the onions and butternut squash. Place them in a large saucepan with the stock, lentils, garlic, cumin, cayenne, and turmeric.

2 Cover and bring to the boil. Reduce the heat and simmer for about 20 to 30 minutes, until the squash and lentils are cooked.

3 Blend the soup until smooth, adding in the coriander, parsley and lemon juice. Add salt and pepper to taste and some water to get the consistency right.

4 Serve garnished with more parsley and coriander.

CHEF'S NOTE

Try also with different kinds of lentils e.g. puy, green or brown.

MATCHA SOUP

260 calories

Ingredients

- 1 red onion, chopped
- 125g/4oz potato, peeled and chopped
- 3 cloves garlic, crushed
- 1 tsp grated fresh ginger
- Pinch cayenne pepper
- Pinch ground black pepper

- 300g/11oz kale, chopped, stems removed
- 1lt/4 cups vegetable stock
- 2 tsp matcha green tea powder
- 1 tbsp chopped fresh coriander/cilantro
- 1 tbsp chopped fresh flat leaf parsley
- 400ml/14floz light coconut milk

Method

1 Put the onion and potato into a large saucepan with a splash of water and cook for 8 minutes, stirring occasionally.

2 Add the garlic, ginger, cayenne and black pepper. Cook for another couple of minutes.

3 Stir in the kale, then add the stock. Bring to the boil, reduce the heat, and simmer covered for half an hour.

4 Stir in the coriander and matcha, and blend until perfectly smooth.

5 Return to the pan, stir in the coconut milk and warm through.

6 Serve with parsley sprinkled over the top.

CHEF'S NOTE
Delicious served with tofu croutons.

WATERCRESS SOUP

182 calories

Ingredients

- 4 garlic cloves
- 300g/11oz potatoes
- 75g/3oz watercress
- 50g/2oz kale
- 2 tbsp extra virgin olive oil
- 1 tsp sea salt
- 1¼lt/5 cups vegetable stock
- 1 tbsp chopped fresh flat leaf parsley
- Pepper, freshly ground
- Lemon wedges to serve

Method

1 Thinly slice the garlic; peel and dice the potatoes. Remove the stems from the watercress and kale and roughly chop.

2 Heat the oil in a large saucepan. Sauté the garlic for about a minute, until fragrant. Stir in the potatoes and half the salt. Cook for another minute.

3 Add the stock and bring to the boil. Reduce the heat and simmer for about 5 minutes.

4 Stir in the watercress and kale. Return to the boil. Reduce to a simmer for 1 more minute. Add the parsley and season with salt and pepper to taste.

5 Serve immediately, and squeeze a lemon wedge into each bowl.

CHEF'S NOTE
This is a chunky unblended soup. Blend if you prefer a smooth texture.

CAULIFLOWER CHEESE SOUP

268 calories

Ingredients

- 1 leek
- 1 red onion
- 2 tbsp extra virgin olive oil
- 300g/11oz cauliflower florets, chopped
- 500ml/2 cups cups semi skimmed milk
- 500ml/2 cups vegetable stock
- 1 bay leaf

- 1 tsp salt
- ½ tsp black pepper
- 2 tbsp buckwheat flour
- 100g/3½oz grated mature cheddar cheese
- 1 tbsp lemon juice
- 3 tbsp chopped chives

Method

1 Wash and thinly slice the leek, discarding the dark green parts. Peel and finely chop the onion.

2 Heat the oil in a large saucepan. Sauté the leek and onion for about five minutes until soft.

3 Add the cauliflower, half the milk, all of the stock, bay leaf, and salt & pepper. Bring to the boil, stirring frequently. Reduce the heat, cover and simmer for 8 to 10 minutes, stirring occasionally, until the cauliflower is tender.

4 Meanwhile, whisk the remaining milk and buckwheat flour in a bowl.

5 Remove the bay leaf from the soup and stir in the buckwheat mixture. Cook over medium heat for another couple of minutes, stirring, until the soup has slightly thickened.

6 Remove the pan from the heat. Stir in the cheese and lemon juice. Serve with chives over the top.

CHEF'S NOTE
If you prefer you can blend this soup for a smooth consistency.

SPLIT PEA AND CELERY SOUP

272 calories

Ingredients

- 8oz/225g green split peas
- 3 celery stalks
- 1 red onion
- 1 clove garlic
- 1lt/4 cups vegetable stock
- 125g/4oz sweet potato
- 2 tbsp chopped flat leaf parsley
- Salt and pepper

Method

1 Wash and drain the peas. Rinse and chop the celery. Peel and chop the onion. Peel and crush the garlic clove.

2 Tip the peas, celery, onion and garlic into a large saucepan. Pour in the stock and cover. Bring to the boil, then reduce the heat and simmer for about 2 hours, stirring occasionally.

3 Peel and dice the sweet potato. Add the sweet potato to the soup and cook for about another half hour until the soup is creamy. Stir in the parsley, season to taste with salt and pepper, and serve adding additional stock or water to get the consistency right.

CHEF'S NOTE

A delicious vegetarian version of traditional pea and ham soup!

GREEN TURNIP SOUP

235 calories

Ingredients

- 1 red onion
- 1 garlic clove
- 300g/11oz turnip
- 150g/5oz sweet potato
- 1lt/4 cups vegetable stock

- 2 large courgettes
- 75g/3oz kale
- 75g/3oz spinach
- 1 tbsp extra virgin olive oil
- Flat leaf parsley or chives to garnish

Method

1 Peel and slice the onion. Peel and crush the garlic. Peel & chop the turnip and the sweet potato. Wash the courgettes, kale and spinach. Chop the courgettes into 1cm slices. Roughly chop the spinach and kale, cutting the thick stems off the kale.

2 Heat the oil in a large saucepan. Sauté the onion and garlic for around 5 minutes, then stir in the turnip and sweet potato, and cook for another 4 or 5 minutes.

3 Pour in the stock and bring to the boil. Reduce the heat and simmer for 10 minutes. Stir in the courgette and kale, and simmer for another 5 minutes. Finally, add the spinach and simmer for another minute or two.

4 Blend the soup until smooth. Adjust the seasoning if necessary, and serve garnished with sprigs of parsley or chives.

CHEF'S NOTE
This is a lovely winter soup. Feel free to add green vegetables that are in season.

HEARTY VEGETABLE SOUP

295 calories

Ingredients

- 2 tbsp extra virgin olive oil
- 2 celery stalks
- 175g/6oz kale
- 1 red onion
- 75g/3oz carrot
- 200g/7oz potato
- 1 garlic clove
- Salt and pepper
- 2 tbsp red wine
- 1lt/4 cups vegetable stock
- 400g/14oz tinned black beans, rinsed and drained

Method

1 Wash and chop the celery and the kale, removing the tough stems from the kale. Peel and chop the onion, carrot and potato. Crush the garlic clove.

2 Heat the oil in a large pan. Sauté the prepared vegetables for around 8 minutes until softened. Add salt & pepper and cook for another minute.

3 Pour in the red wine and vegetable stock. Bring to the boil, reduce the heat, cover, and simmer for 5 minutes.

4 Rinse and drain the beans and add them to the pot. Return to the boil, reduce the heat once more and simmer for another 5 minutes. Serve.

CHEF'S NOTE
Garnish with a sprinkling of Parmesan cheese if desired.

LENTIL AND TOMATO SOUP

300 calories

Ingredients

- 1 tbsp extra virgin olive oil
- 1 red onion, chopped
- 3 celery stalks, chopped
- 800g/1¾lb chopped tinned tomatoes
- 750ml/3 cups vegetable stock
- 300g/11oz dried lentils, rinsed

- 4 tbsp chopped fresh flat leaf parsley
- 120ml/½ cup red wine
- 2 garlic cloves, crushed
- Salt and pepper
- Pinch of ground cloves
- 2 tbsp red wine vinegar

Method

1 Heat the olive oil in a large saucepan, and sauté the onions and celery for about 10 minutes.

2 Pour in the stock, tomatoes and lentils. Bring to the boil. Reduce the heat and simmer, uncovered, for 20 minutes or until the lentils are tender. Remember to stir occasionally.

3 Add the parsley along with the wine, garlic, ground cloves, and seasoning. Simmer for another 20 minutes. Add the red wine vinegar. Simmer another 5 minutes. Serve immediately.

CHEF'S NOTE
You could use balsamic vinegar rather than red wine vinegar.

ROCKET & BROCCOLI SOUP

137 calories

Ingredients

- 1 red onion
- 2 garlic cloves
- 2 tbsp extra virgin olive oil
- 600g/1lb 5oz broccoli

- 1¼lt/5 cups vegetable stock
- Sea salt and black pepper
- 50g/2oz rocket
- 1 lime, sliced into wedges

Method

1 Peel and roughly chop the onion. Thinly slice the garlic cloves. Chop the broccolli..

2 Heat the oil in a large pan. Sauté the onion and garlic for a couple of minutes. Add the broccoli, and cook for 5 more minutes.

3 Add the stock and bring to the boil. Reduce the heat, cover, and simmer for around 10 minutes.

4 Remove the pan from the heat, add the rocket and blend until smooth.

5 Serve the soup garnished with lime wedges.

CHEF'S NOTE
If you prefer, substitute watercress for the rocket.

PURPLE BROCCOLINI SOUP

310 calories

Ingredients

- 200g/7oz purple sprouting broccoli/broccolini
- 4 celery stalks
- 225g/8oz carrots
- 1 red onion
- 1 shallot

- 4 tbsp extra virgin olive oil
- 1lt/4 cups vegetable stock
- 500ml/2 cups milk
- 25g/1oz grated Cheddar cheese
- 2 tbsp crème fraiche

Method

1 Pre-heat the oven to 200 degrees C/400 degrees F/gas mark 6.

2 Rinse the broccoli and celery. Break the broccoli into florets. Roughly chop the celery. Peel and roughly chop the carrots, onion and shallot.

3 Pour about half of the oil into a large roasting tin and add the broccoli. Stir it around until coated in the oil. Season well. Roast in the oven for 25 minutes, or until golden brown.

4 Meanwhile, heat the remaining oil in a large saucepan. Sauté the celery, carrot, onion and shallot with a little salt and pepper for 10 to 12 minutes.

5 Add the roasted broccoli to the pan, pour in the stock and bring to the boil. Reduce the heat and simmer for around 20 minutes or until all the vegetables are soft.

6 Take the pan off the heat and add the milk. Blend the soup until smooth.

7 Serve garnished with a dollop of crème fraiche and a little grated cheese.

CHEF'S NOTE
Serve with a swirl of cream

CAULIFLOWER CURRY SOUP

320 calories

Ingredients

- 1 tbsp extra virgin olive oil
- 1 red onion, chopped
- 1 medium carrot, chopped
- 1 tbsp mild curry powder
- 1 tsp turmeric
- 1 garlic clove, crushed

- 1lt/4 cups vegetable stock
- 125g/4oz potato
- 300g/11oz cauliflower florets
- 400g/14oz tinned chickpeas, drained and rinsed
- 75g/3oz baby kale, chopped

Method

1 Heat the oil in large pan. Sauté the onions and carrots for about 5 minutes. Add the turmeric, curry powder and garlic, and stir well.

2 Cook gently for another couple of minutes and then add the rest of the ingredients. Bring to the boil, reduce the heat and simmer for 15 minutes, or until the vegetables are soft.

3 Blend, season and serve.

CHEF'S NOTE
Enjoy with a spoonful of plain yoghurt.

CHUNKY BUCKWHEAT PASTA SOUP

SERVES 4

357 calories

Ingredients

- 2 tbsp extra virgin olive oil
- 1 red onion, chopped
- 2 garlic cloves, crushed
- 750ml/3 cups vegetable stock
- 100g/3½oz buckwheat pasta
- 75g/3oz carrot, chopped
- 400g/14oz tinned cannellini beans, drained and rinsed
- 225g/8oz kale, roughly chopped, stems removed
- 1 medium courgette, roughly chopped
- 125g/4oz green beans
- 2 tbsp chopped flat leaf parsley
- 50g/2oz grated Parmesan
- 450g/1lb plum tomatoes, peeled and chopped.

Method

1 Heat 1 tbsp of oil in a large pan. Sauté the onion and one of the crushed garlic cloves for around 5 minutes.

2 Pour in the stock and bring to the boil. Add the pasta and the carrot. Cook for 5 minutes. Stir in half the cannellini beans, the kale, courgette and green beans. Bring back to the boil for 5 minutes until the pasta is cooked.

3 Meanwhile blend the remaining beans with the rest of the olive oil, a crushed garlic clove, a tablespoon of water, parsley and cheese.

4 Remove the soup from the heat. Pour in the tomatoes. Stir in the parsley mixture, gently reheat for a minute or two and serve.

CHEF'S NOTE
If you prefer, the parsley blend can be served separate from the soup, or as a garnish. It can be thinned with the addition of more water.

SLOW-COOKED BARLEY AND VEGETABLE SOUP

267 calories

Ingredients

- 150g/5oz parsnips, chopped
- 2 stalks celery, chopped
- 1 clove garlic, chopped
- 1 red onion, chopped
- 200g/7oz turnip, peeled and chopped
- 25g/1oz fresh thyme sprigs, tied together with cotton
- 75g/3oz barley
- 1½ltl/6 cups vegetable stock
- Sea salt and pepper
- 150g/5oz kale, chopped, stems removed
- 4 tsp chopped flat leaf parsley to garnish
- 4 tsp grated Parmesan cheese to garnish

Method

1 Add the the parsnips, celery, garlic, onion, turnip, thyme and barley to your slow cooker, and pour over the stock. Season with salt and pepper. Cover.

2 Cook for 6-7 hours on low. Toward the end of the cooking time (about 15 minutes before you finish cooking) remove the thyme and add the kale. Turn the slow cooker up to high for and continue to cook for a further 15 minutes.

3 Serve garnished generously with parsley, and Parmesan if desired.

CHEF'S NOTE

You can also cook this faster on the high setting for around 4-5 hours, using less stock - about 1lt/4 cups should be enough.

BROCCOLI AND CHEESE SOUP WITH CROUTONS

320 calories

Ingredients

- 1 red onion
- 2 cloves garlic
- 225g/8oz potato
- 2 stalks celery
- 550g/1¼lb broccoli
- 2 slices bread
- 3 tbsp extra virgin olive oil

- Sea salt and pepper
- 750ml/3 cups vegetable stock
- 250ml/1 cup semi skimmed fat milk
- ¼ tsp freshly grated nutmeg
- 175g/6oz mature grated cheddar cheese
- 1 tbsp chopped flat leaf parsley

Method

1 Pre-heat the oven to 400°F/200°C/Gas mark 6

2 Peel and chop the onion, garlic and potatoes. Rinse the celery and broccoli. Chop the celery. Cut the thick stems from the broccoli and chop up the florets.

3 Cube the bread into crouton size pieces and combine with 2 tbsp of the oil. Place on a baking tray and bake for around 6 minutes until crisp and golden. Set aside to cool.

4 Meanwhile, heat the remaining oil in a large pan. Add the onion, celery, garlic, potato and broccoli. Season with salt and pepper and cook, covered, for 5 minutes or so, stirring occasionally, until the vegetables are tender.

5 Pour in the stock, cover and bring to the boil. Reduce the heat and simmer for a couple of minutes until the broccoli is cooked.

6 Remove from heat and blend until smooth. Add the milk and nutmeg and return to the heat for a couple minutes until the soup is warmed through. Add the cheese and stir until melted.

7 Serve with the croutons and garnish with parsley.

CHEF'S NOTE
Use wholemeal bread rather then white bread for the croutons.

SWEET POTATO AND BEAN SOUP

350 calories

Ingredients

- 1 tbsp extra virgin olive oil
- 1 red onion
- 250g/9oz sweet potatoes
- 400g/14oz tinned black beans
- 400g/14oz tinned haricot beans
- 1 tsp crushed garlic

- 1 tsp ground turmeric
- ½ tsp ground coriander/cilantro
- Salt and pepper
- 500ml/2 cups vegetable stock
- 2 tbsp chopped flat leaf parsley
- Juice of 1 lime

Method

1 Peel and chop the onion. Peel and dice the sweet potatoes. Rinse and drain the beans.

2 Heat the oil in a large saucepan over medium heat. Toss in the onion and garlic, and sauté for about 5 minutes until they're soft.

3 Stir in the turmeric and coriander, and season with salt and pepper to taste. Pour in the stock, beans, and diced sweet potatoes. Bring to the boil. Reduce the heat and simmer for around 20 minutes, uncovered, until the potatoes are tender.

4 Pour half of the soup into a large jug and set aside. Blend the rest until smooth then return the blended soup and the contents of the jug into the pan. Stir in the parsley and cook for a few more minutes. Add the lime juice, adjust seasoning to taste and serve.

CHEF'S NOTE
You could also add some buckwheat soup pasta to this dish to turn it into a filling main meal.

LEEK AND POTATO SOUP

320 calories

Ingredients

- 2 tbsp extra virgin olive oil
- 2 medium leeks
- 1 red onion, chopped
- 2 stalks celery, chopped
- 1 medium fennel bulb, chopped
- Sea salt and pepper
- 4 cloves garlic, crushed

- Handful of flat leaf parsley sprigs, tied together with cotton.
- 675g/1½lb potatoes, peeled and diced
- 1½lt/6 cups vegetable stock
- 150g/5oz peas, fresh or frozen
- 1 tbsp fresh lemon juice

Method

1 Heat the oil in a large saucepan. Sauté the chopped leeks, onion, celery stalks and fennel for about 5 minutes. Season with salt and pepper, add the garlic and cook for another 2 minutes.

2 Add the parsley and potatoes, pour in the stock, and bring to the boil. Lower the heat and simmer for 10 minutes stirring occasionally until the potatoes are cooked.

3 Add the peas and cook for another couple of minutes. Remove the parsley sprigs and stir in the lemon juice.

4 Serve garnished with extra fresh parsley.

CHEF'S NOTE
This soup can be frozen for 3 months, but you should freeze it without the lemon juice or additional parsley.

Skinny
SIRT
soup

chilled

VINE TOMATO GAZPACHO

369 calories

Ingredients

- 2 tbsp extra virgin olive oil
- 3 garlic cloves, chopped
- 1 cucumber, halved lengthwise and seeded
- 1 medium avocado, halved and stoned
- 450g/1lb vine ripened tomatoes, chopped
- 1 red pepper, chopped
- 2 bird's eye chillies, de-seeded and chopped
- 500ml/2 cups chicken stock
- 1 tsp brown sugar
- Large pinch sea salt
- 350g/12oz cooked and peeled prawns, chopped
- 50g/2oz green olives, chopped
- 1 red onion, very finely chopped

Method

1 Heat 1 tablespoon of the oil in a small pan. Fry the garlic for a couple of minutes, stirring, until it just begins to brown. Remove from the heat.

2 Coarsely chop half the cucumber and half the avocado and blend with the tomatoes, pepper, chillies and sautéed garlic.

3 When the mixture is smooth, transfer it to a large bowl. Stir in the stock, sugar and salt. Cool and chill.

4 Dice the remaining cucumber and avocado and place in a bowl. Add the shrimp, olives and red onions to make a prawn salad. Drizzle with the remaining tablespoon of oil, and gently toss to combine.

5 To serve, ladle the gazpacho into bowls and top each with some of the prawns salad.

CHEF'S NOTE

For a vegetarian version, use vegetable stock instead of chicken, and leave out the prawns.

CHILLED WATERMELON SOUP

135 calories

Ingredients

- 900g/2lbs finely diced seedless watermelon flesh
- 1 medium cucumber, peeled, seeded and finely diced
- ½ red pepper, finely diced
- 1 tbsp chopped fresh basil
- 2 tbsp chopped flat leaf parsley
- 2 tbsp red wine vinegar
- 1 red onion, chopped
- 1 ½ tbsp extra-virgin olive oil
- Large pinch of salt

Method

1 Mix the watermelon, cucumber, pepper, basil, parsley, vinegar, red onion, olive oil and salt in a large bowl.

2 Remove half the mixture, blend and pour it into a clean bowl.

3 Stir in the remaining diced mixture. Serve either at room temperature, or chilled.

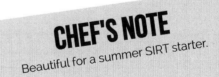

CHEF'S NOTE
Beautiful for a summer SIRT starter.

SPICED CHILLED SOUP

201 calories

Ingredients

- 1 fresh tomato, finely chopped
- ½ red pepper, finely chopped
- ½ green pepper, finely diced
- 1 red onion, finely diced
- ½ cucumber, chopped
- 1 tbsp extra virgin olive oil
- 400g/14oz tinned chopped tomatoes
- 2 garlic cloves, crushed
- 2 bird's eye chillies, de-seeded
- 1½ tsp ground cumin
- ½ tsp ground coriander/cilantro
- 2 tbsp chopped basil
- 2 tbsp chopped flat leaf parsley
- 6 tbsp red wine vinegar
- 1 slice buckwheat rice bread, broken into 4 to 6 pieces
- 500ml/2 cups vegetable juice
- Salt and pepper

Method

1 Keep aside all the tomato, along with enough of the chopped peppers, onion and cucumber for garnish;

2 Place everything else in the blender and season well. Blend until smooth, adjust the seasoning to taste.

3 If you want to alter the alter the consistency of the soup, add a little water.

4 Chill until you are ready to serve it.

5 Garnish with the reserved chopped vegetables.

CHEF'S NOTE
Buckwheat rice bread is available in most health food shops.

74

WALNUT AND STRAWBERRY SOUP

391 calories

Ingredients

- 175g/6oz walnuts, chopped
- 4 slices buckwheat rice bread
- 2 garlic cloves
- 1 tsp salt
- 2 tbsp extra virgin olive oil
- 3 tbsp red wine vinegar
- 1lt/4 cups water
- ½ tsp ground black pepper
- 200g/7oz strawberries, finely diced
- Salt and pepper to season

Method

1 Leave the rice bread in a little water to soften up for a few minutes.

2 Blend the walnuts, soaked bread, garlic and salt with the olive oil, vinegar and the water, until you have a creamy white liquid. Transfer to a bowl.

3 Season to taste with salt and pepper. Cover and refrigerate until well chilled.

4 When you're ready to serve, add the chopped strawberries. Ladle into chilled bowls and serve.

CHEF'S NOTE
Add some freshly chopped chives as a garnish if you wish.

CREAMY BIRD'S EYE SOUP

132 calories

Ingredients

- 1 medium avocado
- 1 red onion
- 2 bird's eye chillies
- 3 tbsp lemon juice
- ½ tsp ground cumin
- 4 plum tomatoes, finely chopped
- Small handful fresh coriander/cilantro
- Small handful rocket
- 1lt/4 cups water
- 3 garlic cloves

Method

1 De-stone and peel the avocado.

2 Peel the onion and de-seed the chillies.

3 Peel the garlic cloves and remove any thick stalks from the fresh herbs.

4 Place everything in the blender and season well. Blend until smooth, adjust the seasoning to taste and serve chilled.

CHEF'S NOTE
You may wish to alter the lemon juice quantity to get the balance right for your own taste.

CELERY AND APPLE SOUP

240 calories

Ingredients

- 4 celery stalks, chopped
- 1 red onion, chopped
- 1 small handful flat leaf parsley
- 1lt/4 cups vegetable stock
- 120ml/½ cup fat free Greek yoghurt
- Sea salt and freshly ground black pepper
- 2 medium apples, peeled, cored & chopped
- 25g/1oz crumbled blue cheese, for garnish

Method

1 Heat the vegetable stock in a large saucepan. Add the apple, celery stalks and their leaves along with the onion and the parsley. Bring to the boil, then turn down the heat and simmer for 10-15 minutes or until the celery is tender.

2 Blend the soup until smooth. Leave to cool to room temperature, then transfer to an airtight container. Refrigerate until well chilled.

3 When the soup is cold and ready to serve, stir in the yoghurt. Season with salt and pepper to taste.

4 Ladle into bowls and garnish with the chopped apple and blue cheese.

CHEF'S NOTE
Celery is a SIRT superfood. Using the leaves in this soup means none of the SIRT goodness goes to waste.

SWEET STRAWBERRY CHILLER

176 calories

Ingredients

- 200g/7oz strawberries
- 125g/4oz cherry tomatoes, chopped
- ½ cucumber, chopped
- 2 bird's eye chillies, de-seeded and chopped
- 1 tbsp fresh chopped mint
- 2 tbsp fresh chopped flat leaf parsley
- Zest and juice from 1 lime
- 3 tbsp honey
- Salt and pepper
- 50g/2oz goat's cheese
- 1 tsp freshly ground black pepper

Method

1 Place all the ingredients, except the goat's cheese, lime zest & black pepper, into a blender and puree until smooth.

2 Pour the soup into a bowl and chill for at least an hour. Stir and adjust the seasoning.

3 Using a fork combine the goat's cheese, lime zest and black pepper in a bowl to make a creamy mixture.

4 Ladle soup into bowls and top with the creamy mixture.

CHEF'S NOTE

Strawberries are an excellent source of vitamin C and K.

COOL GREEN SOUP

198
calories

Ingredients

- 2 tbsp extra virgin olive oil
- 1 red onion, chopped
- 1 carrot, peeled & finely chopped
- 2 celery stalks, sliced
- 1.5l/6 cups chicken stock
- 75g/3oz uncooked rice

- 300g/11oz fresh spinach, chopped
- Small handful of shredded lettuce
- Large bunch flat leaf parsley
- Salt and black pepper
- 1 pinch cayenne pepper

Method

1 Heat the olive oil in a large saucepan. Sauté the onion, carrot, and celery for about 5 minutes, until the onion has softened.

2 Add the chicken stock and rice, and bring to the boil. Cover the soup, lower the heat and simmer for 35 minutes until the rice is cooked.

3 Stir in the spinach, lettuce, and parsley. Cook for about 5 minutes until wilted. Season with salt, black pepper and cayenne pepper.

4 Blend the soup until smooth. Alter the consistency if you wish by adding a little more stock. Chill and serve.

CHEF'S NOTE
Chopped raw walnuts make a great garnish for this chilled soup.

SERVES 4

FRESH CORN & CAYENNE SOUP

260 calories

Ingredients

- 200g/7oz ripe tomatoes
- 3 fresh sweet corn cobs, kernels removed
- 2 yellow peppers, de-seeded & chopped
- 1 garlic clove, crushed
- Large pinch cayenne pepper
- ½ tsp salt
- 2 tbsp white wine vinegar
- 2 tbsp extra virgin olive oil
- 1 red onion, finely chopped, to garnish
- 1 avocado
- 25g/1oz walnut
- 1 bird's eye chilli, de-seeded

Method

1 Add all the ingredients, except the avocado, walnuts & chilli into a blender.

2 Blend until smooth and adjust the seasoning to taste.

3 Refrigerate until properly chilled.

4 Whilst the soup is chilling prepare the fresh garnish by de-stoning and chopping the avocado flesh. Finely chop the walnuts & chilli and combine with the avocado.

5 When you're ready to serve, pour the soup into bowls. Garnish with the fresh avocado mixture and serve.

CHEF'S NOTE
Feel fee to use tinned sweet corn if you don't have time to remove the kernels from fresh sweet corn ears.

80

Skinny
SIRT
soup

fruit

MELON, PINEAPPLE & PEACH SOUP

280 calories

Ingredients

- ½ cantaloupe melon, seeds removed, peeled, roughly chopped
- 200g/7oz fresh pineapple, roughly chopped
- 2 medium peaches peeled, stoned, chopped
- 1 medium apple, cored, peeled & chopped
- 200g/7oz strawberries, halved
- 2 tsp brown sugar
- 1 tbsp honey
- 1lt/4 cups water
- 4 tbsp low fat crème fraiche

Method

1 Combine all the prepared fruit in a large saucepan. Mix in the sugar and honey. Pour in the water and gently simmer for about 10-15 minutes.

2 Allow the fruit to cool. Place in a blender and puree until smooth. Chill in the fridge until ready to serve.

3 Spoon into bowls, and garnish with a dollop of crème fraiche.

CHEF'S NOTE
Cantaloupe melon is a good source of vitamin B6, niacin and folate.

GINGER & PINEAPPLE SOUP

170 calories

Ingredients

- 1 tbsp extra virgin olive oil
- 1 tsp fresh grated ginger
- 300g/11oz strawberries, halved
- 200g/7oz pineapple, chopped
- 125g/4oz mango, chopped
- 500ml/2 cups water
- 2 tbsp brown sugar
- 2 tbsp lemon juice
- 50g/2oz blueberries
- 1 tbsp chopped mint

Method

1 Heat the oil and gently sauté the ginger in a large saucepan for a few minutes.

2 Add the fruit and cook for a few minutes. Add the water, sugar & lemon juice.

3 Increase the heat and simmer for 5 minutes.

4 Allow the soup to cool and then blend until smooth.

5 Cover, chill and serve with fresh mint sprinkled over the top.

CHEF'S NOTE
Ginger helps eliminate unwanted gases from the digestive system and soothes the intestinal tract.

BLACKBERRY & RED WINE SOUP

180 calories

Ingredients

- 175g/6oz cantaloupe melon, de-seeded & cubed
- 125g/4oz blackberries
- 500ml/2 cups pomegranate juice
- 250ml/1 cup water
- 120ml/½ cup red wine
- 2 tbsp fresh lemon juice
- 1 tbsp honey
- 200g/7oz strawberries, finely chopped
- 1 tbsp chopped mint

Method

1 In a blender, puree the melon, blackberries, pomegranate juice, water, red wine, honey & lemon juice until smooth.

2 Allow the soup to chill.

3 Divide into bowls. Garnish with finely chopped tomatoes and a little fresh mint. Pour soup into a container, cover, and chill for at least 1 hour, or up to 1 day.

4 Pour the soup into shallow bowls. Scatter the sliced strawberries on top.

CHEF'S NOTE
Red wine contains resveratrol which is thought help keep the heart healthy.

CHUNKY YOGHURT FRUIT SOUP

290 calories

Ingredients

- 450g/1lb honeydew melon
- 200g/7oz strawberries
- 500ml/2 cups fat free Greek yoghurt
- 120ml/½ cup fresh orange juice

- 1 tbsp lemon juice
- 1 tbsp crushed crystalized ginger
- 1 tbsp chopped mint

Method

1 De-seed the melon and cube.

2 Remove any green tops from the strawberries and slice.

3 Combine all the ingredients together in a large bowl and chill for at least an hour.

4 Divide into bowls and serve garnished with some chopped mint.

CHEF'S NOTE
The high water content and potassium levels make honeydew lemon effective in maintaining healthy blood pressure levels.

BUCKWHEAT STRAWBERRY 'SOUP'

330 calories

Ingredients

- 800g/1¾lb strawberries
- 1lt/4 cups soya milk
- 2 tbsp chopped mint
- 2 tbsp chopped walnuts
- 1 tbsp buckwheat flakes

Method

1 Remove any green tops from the strawberries and chop.

2 Blend the strawberries together with the soya milk.

3 Serve in bowls with the chopped mint, walnuts and buckwheat flakes sprinkled over the top.

CHEF'S NOTE
Also known as groats, buckwheat flakes are a great SIRT ingredient.

AROMATIC BUCKWHEAT FRUIT SOUP

370 calories

Ingredients

- 200g/7oz red grapes, halved
- 1 orange, peeled and chopped
- ½ banana, mashed
- 60ml/¼ cup single cream
- 60ml/¼ cup fat free Greek yoghurt
- 180ml/¾ cup skimmed milk
- 120ml/½ cup orange juice
- 50g/2oz buckwheat flour
- 120ml/ ½ cup cold water
- 2 tbsp honey
- 2 tsp ground cinnamon
- ½ tsp ground nutmeg
- ¾tsp nutmeg
- 100g/3½oz strawberries, sliced
- 100g/3½oz blueberries

Method

1 Add the grapes, orange, banana, cream, yoghurt, milk & orange juice to a large saucepan and gently cook on a low heat.

2 Meanwhile, blend the buckwheat flour and water together to create a smooth paste.

3 Continue to cook the fruit on a medium heat for about 5 minutes, stirring occasionally.

4 Add the buckwheat paste, lower the heat, cover and simmer for another 3 minutes stirring occasionally.

5 Serve warm, garnished with the sliced strawberries and blueberries.

CHEF'S NOTE
Cinnamon helps reduce the rise in blood sugar after eating.

NO-COOK WALNUT & ORANGE SOUP

SERVES 4

145 calories

Ingredients

- 500ml/2 cups orange juice
- 60ml/ ¼ cup fat free Greek yoghurt
- 1 tbsp honey
- 2 tsp lemon juice
- 1 small banana, sliced

- 125g/4oz raspberries
- 100g/3½oz strawberries
- 100g/3½oz blueberries
- 50g/2oz walnuts, chopped

Method

1 In a mixing bowl, whisk together the orange juice, yoghurt, honey and lemon juice.

2 Divide the sliced banana and berries evenly between 4 bowls and pour the orange juice mixture over the top.

3 Sprinkle the chopped walnuts over the soup and serve.

CHEF'S NOTE
Walnuts are a good source of protein, fibre and healthy fats.

CINNAMON & APPLE JUICE SOUP

220 calories

Ingredients

- 200g/7oz strawberries
- 125g/4oz berries (blueberries, blackberries & raspberries)
- 750ml/3 cups apple juice
- 1 cinnamon stick
- 2 whole cloves
- 1 tbsp buckwheat flour
- 1 tsp vanilla essence
- 4 tbsp sour cream
- Small handful fresh mint, chopped

Method

1 In a saucepan, combine the berries, half the apple juice, cinnamon, and cloves. Bring to the boil, lower the heat and simmer, uncovered, for 8-10 minutes, stirring occasionally.

2 In a separate bowl, stir the buckwheat flour into the remaining apple juice until you have got a smooth paste. Add it to the pan and continue cooking for a few minutes until the soup is slightly thickened.

3 Remove the pan from heat and stir in the vanilla. Discard the cinnamon stick and the cloves.

4 Divide the soup into bowl and garnish with a dollop of sour cream along with a little chopped mint.

CHEF'S NOTE
Mint has positive anti-bacterial & anti-inflammatory properties which makes it great for oral health.

Other COOKNATION TITLES

If you enjoyed **The Skinny Sirtfood Soup Recipe Book** we'd really appreciate your feedback. Reviews help others decide if this is the right book for them so a moment of your time would be appreciated.

Thank you.

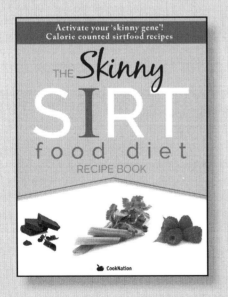

You may also be interested in:

The Skinny Sirtfood Diet Recipe Book: Activate your 'skinny gene'! Calorie counted sirtfood recipes.

To browse our full catalogue visit **www.bellmackenzie.com**

Printed in Great Britain
by Amazon